Deliciously

Keto Vegetarian

Lose Weight &
Increase your Energy
with Easy and Tasty Recipes

Ricardo Abagnale

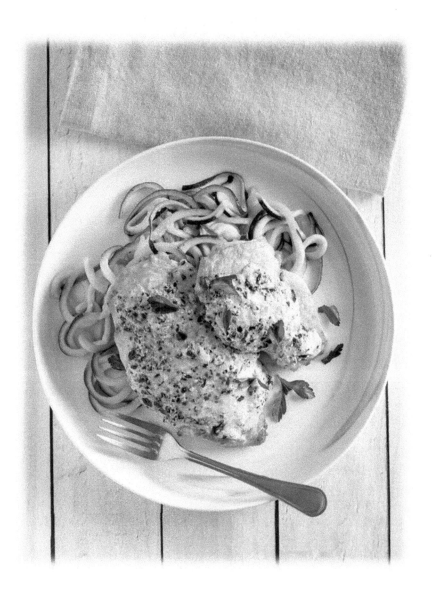

Table of Contents

INTRODUCTION **6**

BREAKFAST **7**

    SWEET CAULIFLOWER RICE CASSEROLE 7

    SPICY BOWLS 9

    KETO PUMPKIN PANCAKES 11

MAINS **13**

    ARUGULA AND ARTICHOKES BOWLS 13

    MINTY ARUGULA SOUP 15

    SPINACH AND BROCCOLI SOUP 17

    COCONUT ZUCCHINI CREAM 19

    ZUCCHINI AND CAULIFLOWER SOUP 21

    CHARD SOUP 23

    AVOCADO, PINE NUTS AND CHARD SALAD 25

    GRAPES, AVOCADO AND SPINACH SALAD 27

SIDES **29**

    CREAMY CAJUN ZUCCHINIS 29

    HERBED ZUCCHINIS AND OLIVES 31

    VEGGIE PAN 33

    MASALA BRUSSELS SPROUTS 35

    NUTMEG GREEN BEANS 37

    PEPPERS AND CELERY SAUTÉ 39

FRUIT AND VEGETABLES **41**

    SMOKY COLESLAW 41

    SIMPLE SESAME STIR-FRY 43

    MEDITERRANEAN HUMMUS PIZZA 46

    BAKED BRUSSELS SPROUTS 48

MINTED PEAS 50

EDAMAME DONBURI 52

SOUPS AND STEWS 54

ITALIAN WEDDING SOUP 54

ROASTED VEGETABLE BISQUE 57

SPICY GAZPACHO 59

KETO PASTA 61

PARSLEY-LIME PASTA.. 61

SALADS 64

RICE SALAD WITH CASHEWS AND DRIED PAPAYA 64

SPINACH SALAD WITH ORANGE-DIJON DRESSING 66

CARAMELIZED ONION AND BEET SALAD 68

TREASURE BARLEY SALAD 71

SNACKS 73

GARDEN SALAD WRAPS 73

BLACK SESAME WONTON CHIPS 75

MARINATED MUSHROOM WRAPS 77

TAMARI TOASTED ALMONDS.. 79

AVOCADO AND TEMPEH BACON WRAPS 81

DESSERTS 83

CHERRY-VANILLA RICE PUDDING (PRESSURE COOKER) 83

CHOCOLATE COCONUT BROWNIES...85

LIME IN THE COCONUT CHIA PUDDING...87

STRAWBERRY PARFAITS WITH CASHEW CRÈME 89

MINT CHOCOLATE CHIP SORBET 91

PEACH-MANGO CRUMBLE (PRESSURE COOKER) 93

GINGER-SPICE BROWNIES 96

CHOCOLATE AND WALNUT FARFALLE 98

ALMOND-DATE ENERGY BITES 100

OTHER RECIPES **102**

CLOUD BREAD 102

FATHEAD CRACKERS..104

QUESO BLANCO DIP..106

CLASSIC BUTTERMILK SYRUP..108

BAKED ONION RINGS... 110

INTRODUCTION

The Ketogenic diet is truly life changing. The diet improves your overall health and helps you lose the extra weight in a matter of days. The diet will show its multiple benefits even from the beginning and it will become your new lifestyle really soon.

As soon as you embrace the Ketogenic diet, you will start to live a completely new life.

On the other hand, the vegetarian diet is such a healthy dietary option you can choose when trying to live healthy and also lose some weight.

The collection we bring to you today is actually a combination between the Ketogenic and vegetarian diets. You get to discover some amazing Ketogenic vegetarian dishes you can prepare in the comfort of your own home. All the dishes you found here follow both the Ketogenic and the vegetarian rules, they all taste delicious and rich and they are all easy to make.

We can assure you that such a combo is hard to find. So, start a keto diet with a vegetarian "touch" today. It will be both useful and fun!

So, what are you still waiting for? Get started with the Ketogenic diet and learn how to prepare the best and most flavored Ketogenic vegetarian dishes. Enjoy them all!

Sweet Cauliflower Rice Casserole

Preparation time: 10 minutes

Cooking time: 1 hour

Servings: 8

Nutritional Values (Per Serving):

- Calories 213
- Fat 4.1
- Fiber 4
- Carbs 41
- Protein 4.5

Ingredients:

- 1 and ½ cups blackberries
- 1 cup coconut cream
- 1 tablespoon cinnamon powder
- 2 teaspoons vanilla extract
- 1 teaspoon ginger, ground

- 1 cup cauliflower rice
- ¼ cup walnuts, chopped
- 2 cups almond milk

Directions:

1. In a baking dish, combine the cauliflower rice with the berries, the cream and the other ingredients, toss and bake at 350 degrees F for 1 hour.
2. Divide the mix into bowls and serve for breakfast.

Spicy Bowls

Preparation time: 10 minutes

Cooking time: 15 minutes

Servings: 4

Nutritional Values (Per Serving):

- Calories 116
- Fat 11.3
- Fiber 1.6
- Carbs 4.2
- Protein 1.3

Ingredients:

- 1 cup baby spinach
- ½ cup cherry tomatoes, halved
- ¼ teaspoon cardamom, ground
- 1 teaspoon turmeric powder
- 1 tablespoon olive oil
- A pinch of salt and black pepper
- ½ cup coconut cream
- ½ cup green olives, pitted and halved

- ½ cup cucumbers, sliced
- 1 tablespoon parsley, chopped

Directions:
1. Heat up a pan with the oil over medium heat, add the olives and the tomatoes, toss and cook for 5 minutes.
2. Add the spinach and the other ingredients, toss, cook over medium heat fro 10 minutes, divide into bowls and serve.

Keto Pumpkin Pancakes

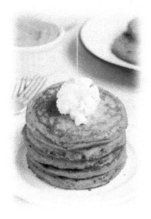

Preparation time: 10 minutes

Cooking time: 6 minutes

Servings: 8

Nutritional Values (Per Serving):

- Calories: 150
- Fat: 11 g
- Carbs: 1.5 g
- Protein: 5.5 g

Ingredients:

- 2 tablespoons butter
- 1 teaspoon pumpkin spice

- 1 teaspoon baking powder
- 2 large eggs
- ¼ cup sour cream
- 1 cup almond meal
- ¼ cup pumpkin puree
- 1/4 teaspoon salt

Directions:

1. First in a mixing bowl combine your eggs, sour cream and butter. In another mixing bowl, combine salt, almond meal, spice, baking powder. Now slowly add your wet ingredients to your dry ingredients, while stirring to blend. This will give you a sweet, smooth batter.

2. Over medium-heat warm up a cast- iron frying pan and grease it with butter. Pour about 1/3 of your mixture into the skillet. When bubbles begin to form on top of the batter, allow it to cook for about another minute, then flip it over. Cook on the other side for an additional minute or so.

3. Repeat the previous last two steps until your batter is done. Serve up your keto pumpkin pancakes with your favorite toppings.

Arugula and Artichokes Bowls

Preparation time: 5 minutes

Cooking time: 0 minutes

Servings: 4

Nutritional Values (Per Serving):

- Calories 200
- Fat 2
- Fiber 1
- Carbs 5
- Protein 7

Ingredients:

- 2 cups baby arugula
- ¼ cup walnuts, chopped
- 1 cup canned artichoke hearts, drained and quartered

- 1 tablespoon balsamic vinegar
- 2 tablespoons cilantro, chopped
- 2 tablespoons olive oil
- Salt and black pepper to the taste
- 1 tablespoon lemon juice

Directions:

1. In a bowl, combine the artichokes with the arugula, walnuts and the other ingredients, toss, divide into smaller bowls and serve for lunch.

Minty Arugula Soup

Preparation time: 5 minutes

Cooking time: 10 minutes

Servings: 4

Nutritional Values (Per Serving):

- Calories 200
- Fat 4
- Fiber 2
- Carbs 6
- Protein 10

Ingredients:

- 3 scallions, chopped
- 1 tablespoon olive oil
- ½ cup coconut milk
- 2 cups baby arugula
- 2 tablespoons mint, chopped

- 6 cups vegetable stock
- 2 tablespoons chives, chopped
- Salt and black pepper to the taste

Directions:

1. Heat up a pot with the oil over medium high heat, add the scallions and sauté for 2 minutes.
2. Add the rest of the ingredients, toss, bring to a simmer and cook over medium heat for 8 minutes more.
3. Divide the soup into bowls and serve.

Spinach and Broccoli Soup

Preparation time: 10 minutes

Cooking time: 20 minutes

Servings: 4

Nutritional Values (Per Serving):

- Calories 150
- Fat 3
- Fiber 1
- Carbs 3
- Protein 7

Ingredients:

- 3 shallots, chopped
- 1 tablespoon olive oil
- 2 garlic cloves, minced
- ½ pound broccoli florets
- ½ pound baby spinach

- Salt and black pepper to the taste
- 4 cups veggie stock
- 1 teaspoon turmeric powder
- 1 tablespoon lime juice

Directions:

1. Heat up a pot with the oil over medium high heat, add the shallots and the garlic and sauté for 5 minutes.
2. Add the broccoli, spinach and the other ingredients, toss, bring to a simmer and cook over medium heat for 15 minutes.
3. Ladle into soup bowls and serve.

Coconut Zucchini Cream

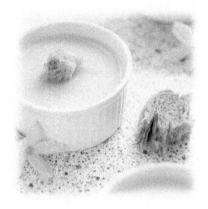

Preparation time: 10 minutes

Cooking time: 25 minutes

Servings: 4

Nutritional Values (Per Serving):

- Calories 160
- Fat 4
- Fiber 2
- Carbs 4
- Protein 8

Ingredients:

- 1 pound zucchinis, roughly chopped
- 2 tablespoons avocado oil
- 4 scallions, chopped
- Salt and black pepper to the taste
- 6 cups veggie stock
- 1 teaspoon basil, dried
- 1 teaspoon cumin, ground
- 3 garlic cloves, minced
- ¾ cup coconut cream
- 1 tablespoon dill, chopped

Directions:

1. Heat up a pot with the oil over medium high heat, add the scallions and the garlic and sauté for 5 minutes.
2. Add the rest of the ingredients, stir, bring to a simmer and cook over medium heat for 20 minutes more.
3. Blend the soup using an immersion blender, ladle into bowls and serve.

Zucchini and Cauliflower Soup

Preparation time: 10 minutes

Cooking time: 25 minutes

Servings: 4

Nutritional Values (Per Serving):

- Calories 154
- Fat 12
- Fiber 3
- Carbs 5
- Protein 4

Ingredients:

- 4 scallions, chopped
- 1 teaspoon ginger, grated
- 2 tablespoons olive oil
- 1 pound zucchinis, sliced
- 2 cups cauliflower florets

- Salt and black pepper to the taste
- 6 cups veggie stock
- 1 garlic clove, minced
- 1 tablespoon lemon juice
- 1 cup coconut cream

Directions:

1. Heat up a pot with the oil over medium heat, add the scallions, ginger and the garlic and sauté for 5 minutes.
2. Add the rest of the ingredients, bring to a simmer and cook over medium heat for 20 minutes.
3. Blend everything using an immersion blender, ladle into soup bowls and serve.

Chard Soup

Preparation time: 10 minutes

Cooking time: 25 minutes

Servings: 4

Nutritional Values (Per Serving):

- Calories 232
- Fat 23
- Fiber 3
- Carbs 4
- Protein 3

Ingredients:

- 1 pound Swiss chard, chopped
- ½ cup shallots, chopped
- 1 tablespoon avocado oil
- 1 teaspoon cumin, ground
- 1 teaspoon rosemary, dried

- 1 teaspoon basil, dried
- 2 garlic cloves, minced
- Salt and black pepper to the taste
- 6 cups vegetable stock
- 1 tablespoon tomato passata
- 1 tablespoon cilantro, chopped

Directions:

1. Heat up a pan with the oil over medium heat, add the shallots and the garlic and sauté for 5 minutes.
2. Add the Swiss chard and the other ingredients, toss, bring to a simmer and cook over medium heat for 20 minutes more.
3. Divide the soup into bowls and serve.

Avocado, Pine Nuts and Chard Salad

Preparation time: 5 minutes

Cooking time: 15 minutes

Servings: 4

Nutritional Values (Per Serving):

- Calories 120
- Fat 2
- Fiber 1
- Carbs 4
- Protein 8

Ingredients:

- 1 pound Swiss chard, roughly chopped
- 2 tablespoons olive oil
- 1 avocado, peeled, pitted and roughly cubed

- 2 spring onions, chopped
- ¼ cup pine nuts, toasted
- 1 tablespoon balsamic vinegar
- Salt and black pepper to the taste

Directions:

1. Heat up a pan with the oil over medium heat, add the spring onions, pine nuts and the chard, stir and sauté for 5 minutes.
2. Add the vinegar and the other ingredients, toss, cook over medium heat for 10 minutes more, divide into bowls and serve for lunch.

Grapes, Avocado and Spinach Salad

Preparation time: 10 minutes

Cooking time: 0 minutes

Servings: 4

Nutritional Values (Per Serving):

- Calories 190
- Fat 17.1
- Fiber 4.6
- Carbs 10.9
- Protein 1.7

Ingredients:

- 1 cup green grapes, halved
- 2 cups baby spinach
- 1 avocado, pitted, peeled and cubed

- Salt and black pepper to the taste
- 2 tablespoons olive oil
- 1 tablespoon thyme, chopped
- 1 tablespoon rosemary, chopped
- 1 tablespoon lime juice
- 1 garlic clove, minced

Directions:

1. In a salad bowl, combine the grapes with the spinach and the other ingredients, toss, and serve for lunch.

Creamy Cajun Zucchinis

Preparation time: 10 minutes

Cooking time: 20 minutes

Servings: 4

Nutritional Values (Per Serving):

- Calories 200
- Fat 2
- Fiber 1
- Carbs 5
- Protein 8

Ingredients:

- 1 pound zucchinis, roughly cubed
- 2 tablespoons olive oil
- 4 scallions, chopped

- Salt and black pepper to the taste
- 1 teaspoon Cajun seasoning
- A pinch of cayenne pepper
- 1 cup coconut cream
- 1 tablespoon dill, chopped

Directions:

- Heat up a pan with the oil over medium heat, add the scallions, cayenne and Cajun seasoning, stir and sauté for 5 minutes.
- Add the zucchinis and the other ingredients, toss, cook over medium heat for 15 minutes more, divide between plates and serve.

Herbed Zucchinis and Olives

Preparation time: 10 minutes

Cooking time: 20 minutes

Servings: 4

Nutritional Values (Per Serving):

- Calories 200
- Fat 20
- Fiber 4
- Carbs 3
- Protein 1

Ingredients:

- 1 cup kalamata olives, pitted
- 1 cup green olives, pitted
- 1 pound zucchinis, roughly cubed
- 1 tablespoon rosemary, chopped
- 1 tablespoon basil, chopped

- 1 tablespoon cilantro, chopped
- 2 tablespoons olive oil
- 3 garlic cloves, minced
- 1 tablespoon lemon juice
- 1 teaspoon lemon zest, grated
- 1 tablespoon sweet paprika
- A pinch of salt and black pepper

Directions:

1. Heat up a pan with the oil over medium heat, add the garlic, lemon zest and paprika and sauté for 2 minutes.
2. Add the olives, zucchinis and the other ingredients, toss, cook over medium heat for 18 minutes more, divide between plates and serve.

Veggie Pan

Preparation time: 10 minutes

Cooking time: 20 minutes

Servings: 4

Nutritional Values (Per Serving):

- Calories 137
- Fat 7.7
- Fiber 7.1
- Carbs 18.1
- Protein 3.4

Ingredients:

- 1 cup green beans, trimmed and halved
- 1 cup cherry tomatoes, halved
- 1 zucchini, roughly cubed
- 1 red bell pepper, cut into strips
- 1 eggplant, cubed

- 3 scallions, chopped
- 2 tablespoons olive oil
- 2 tablespoons lime juice
- Salt and black pepper to the taste
- 1 teaspoon chili powder
- 1 tablespoon cilantro, chopped
- 3 garlic cloves, minced

Directions:

1. Heat up a pan with the oil over medium heat, add the scallions, chili powder and the garlic and sauté for 5 minutes.
2. Add the green beans, tomatoes and the other ingredients, toss, cook over medium heat for 15 minutes.
3. Divide the mix between plates and serve as a side dish.

Masala Brussels Sprouts

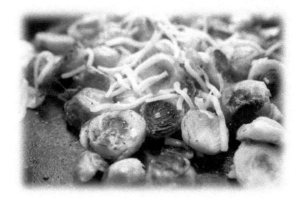

Preparation time: 10 minutes

Cooking time: 35 minutes

Servings: 4

Nutritional Values (Per Serving):

- Calories 115
- Fat 7.6
- Fiber 4.9
- Carbs 11.2
- Protein 4.2

Ingredients:

- 1 pound Brussels sprouts, trimmed and halved
- Salt and black pepper to the taste
- 1 tablespoon garam masala
- 2 tablespoons olive oil
- 1 tablespoon caraway seeds

Directions:

1. In a roasting pan, combine the sprouts with the masala and the other ingredients, toss and bake at 400 degrees F for 35 minutes.
2. Divide the mix between plates and serve.

Nutmeg Green Beans

Preparation time: 10 minutes

Cooking time: 30 minutes

Servings: 4

Nutritional Values (Per Serving):

- Calories 100
- Fat 13
- Fibe
- 2.3
- Carbs 5.1
- Protein 2

Ingredients:

- 2 tablespoons olive oil
- ½ cup coconut cream
- 1 pound green beans, trimmed and halved
- 1 teaspoon nutmeg, ground

- A pinch of salt and cayenne pepper
- ½ teaspoon onion powder
- ½ teaspoon garlic powder
- 2 tablespoons parsley, chopped

Directions:

1. Heat up a pan with the oil over medium heat, add the green beans, nutmeg and the other ingredients, toss, cook for 30 minutes, divide the mix between plates and serve.

Peppers and Celery Sauté

Preparation time: 10 minutes

Cooking time: 15 minutes

Servings: 4

Nutritional Values (Per Serving):

- Calories 87
- Fat 2.4
- Fiber 3
- Carbs 5
- Protein 4

Ingredients:

- 1 red bell pepper, cut into medium chunks
- 1 green bell pepper, cut into medium chunks
- 1 celery stalk, chopped
- 2 scallions, chopped
- 2 tablespoons olive oil

- Salt and black pepper to the taste
- 1 tablespoons parsley, chopped
- 1 teaspoon cumin, ground
- 2 garlic cloves, minced

Directions:

1. Heat up a pan with the oil over medium heat, add the scallions, garlic and cumin and sauté for 5 minutes.
2. Add the peppers, celery and the other ingredients, toss, cook over medium heat for 10 minutes more, divide between plates and serve.

Smoky Coleslaw

Preparation time: 10 minutes

Cooking time: 0 minutes

Servings: 6

Nutritional Values (Per Serving):

- Calories: 73
- Fat: 4g
- Protein: 1g
- Carbohydrates: 8g
- . Fiber: 2g
- Sugar: 5g
- Sodium: 283mg

Ingredients:

- 1 pound shredded cabbage

- ⅓ cup vegan mayonnaise
- ¼ cup unseasoned rice vinegar
- 3 tablespoons plain vegan yogurt or plain soymilk
- 1 tablespoon vegan sugar
- ½ teaspoon salt
- ¼ teaspoon freshly ground black pepper
- ¼ teaspoon smoked paprika
- ¼ teaspoon chipotle powder

Directions:

1. Put the shredded cabbage in a large bowl. In a medium bowl, whisk the mayonnaise, vinegar, yogurt, sugar, salt, pepper, paprika, and chipotle powder.
2. Pour over the cabbage, and mix with a spoon or spatula and until the cabbage shreds are coated. Divide the coleslaw evenly among 6 single-serving containers. Seal the lids.

Simple Sesame Stir-Fry

Preparation time: 10 minutes

Cooking time: 20 minutes

Servings: 4

Nutritional Values (Per Serving):

- Calories: 334
- Total fat: 13g
- Carbs: 42g
- Fiber: 9g
- Protein: 17g

Ingredients:

- 1 cup quinoa
- 2 cups water Pinch sea salt
- 1 head broccoli
- 1 to 2 teaspoons untoasted sesame oil, or olive oil

- 1 cup snow peas, or snap peas, ends trimmed and cut in half
- 1 cup frozen shelled edamame beans, or peas
- 2 cups chopped Swiss chard, or other large-leafed green 2 scallions, chopped
- 2 tablespoons water
- 1 teaspoon toasted sesame oil
- 1 tablespoon tamari, or soy sauce
- 2 tablespoons sesame seeds

Directions:

1. Put the quinoa, water, and sea salt in a medium pot, bring it to a boil for a minute, then turn to low and simmer, covered, for 20 minutes. The quinoa is fully cooked when you see the swirl of the grains with a translucent center, and it is fluffy. Do not stir the quinoa while it is cooking.

2. Meanwhile, cut the broccoli into bite-size florets, cutting and pulling apart from the stem. Also chop the stem into bite-size pieces. Heat a large skillet to high, and sauté the broccoli in the untoasted sesame oil, with a pinch of salt to help it soften. Keep this moving continuously, so that it doesn't burn, and add an extra drizzle of oil if needed as you add the rest of the vegetables. Add the snow peas

next, continuing to stir. Add the edamame until they thaw. Add the Swiss chard and scallions at the same time, tossing for only a minute to wilt. Then add 2 tablespoons of water to the hot skillet so that it sizzles and finishes the vegetables with a quick steam.

3. Dress with the toasted sesame oil and tamari, and toss one last time. Remove from the heat immediately. Serve a scoop of cooked quinoa, topped with stir-fry and sprinkled with some sesame seeds, and an extra drizzle of tamari and/or toasted sesame oil if you like.

Mediterranean Hummus Pizza

Preparation time: 10 minutes

Cooking time: 30 minutes

Servings: 2 pizzas

Nutrition (1 pizza):

- Calories: 500
- Total fat: 25g
- Carbs: 58g
- Fiber: 12g
- Protein: 19g

Ingredients:

- ½ zucchini, thinly sliced
- ½ red onion, thinly sliced
- 1 cup cherry tomatoes, halved
- 2 to 4 tablespoons pitted and chopped black olives
- Pinch sea salt

- Drizzle olive oil (optional)
- 2 prebaked pizza crusts
- ½ cup Classic Hummus, or Roasted Red Pepper Hummus 2 to 4 tablespoons Cheesy Sprinkle

Directions:

1. Preheat the oven to 400°F. Place the zucchini, onion, cherry tomatoes, and olives in a large bowl, sprinkle them with the sea salt, and toss them a bit. Drizzle with a bit of olive oil (if using), to seal in the flavor and keep them from drying out in the oven.
2. Lay the two crusts out on a large baking sheet. Spread half the hummus on each crust, and top with the veggie mixture and some Cheesy Sprinkle. Pop the pizzas in the oven for 20 to 30 minutes, or until the veggies are soft.

Baked Brussels Sprouts

Preparation time: 10 minutes

Cooking time: 40 minutes

Servings: 4

Nutritional Values (Per Serving):

- Calories: 77
- Fat: 3g
- Protein: 4g
- Carbohydrates: 12g
- Fiber: 5g
- Sugar: 3g
- Sodium: 320mg

Ingredients:

- 1 pound Brussels sprouts
- 2 teaspoons extra-virgin olive or canola oil
- 4 teaspoons minced garlic (about 4 cloves)

- 1 teaspoon dried oregano
- ½ teaspoon dried rosemary
- ½ teaspoon salt
- ¼ teaspoon freshly ground black pepper
- 1 tablespoon balsamic vinegar

Directions:

1. Preheat the oven to 400°F. Line a rimmed baking sheet with parchment paper. Trim and halve the Brussels sprouts. Transfer to a large bowl. Toss with the olive oil, garlic, oregano, rosemary, salt, and pepper to coat well.
2. Transfer to the prepared baking sheet. Bake for 35 to 40 minutes, shaking the pan occasionally to help with even browning, until crisp on the outside and tender on the inside. Remove from the oven and transfer to a large bowl. Stir in the balsamic vinegar, coating well.
3. Divide the Brussels sprouts evenly among 4 single-serving containers. Let cool before sealing the lids.

Minted Peas

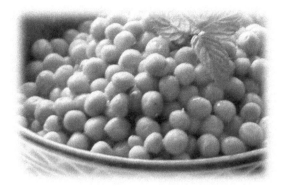

Preparation time: 5 minutes

Cooking time: 5 minutes

Servings: 4

Ingredients:

- 1 tablespoon olive oil
- 4 cups peas, fresh or frozen (not canned
- ½ teaspoon sea salt
- freshly ground black pepper
- 3 tablespoons chopped fresh mint

Directions:

- In a large sauté pan, heat the olive oil over medium-high heat until hot. Add the peas and cook, about 5 minutes.
- Remove the pan from heat. Stir in the salt, season with pepper, and stir in the mint.
- Serve hot.

Edamame Donburi

Preparation time: 5 minutes

Cooking time: 20 minutes

Servings: 4

Ingredients:

- 1 cup fresh or frozen shelled edamame
- 1 tablespoon canola or grapeseed oil
- 1 medium yellow onion, minced
- 5 shiitake mushroom caps, lightly rinsed, patted dry, and cut into 1/4-inch strips
- 1 teaspoon grated fresh ginger
- 3 green onions, minced
- 8 ounces firm tofu, drained and crumbled
- 2 tablespoons soy sauce
- 3 cups hot cooked white or brown rice
- 1 tablespoon toasted sesame oil
- 1 tablespoon toasted sesame seeds, for garnish

Directions:

1. In a small saucepan of boiling salted water, cook the edamame until tender, about 10 minutes. Drain and set aside.

2. In a large skillet, heat the canola oil over medium heat. Add the onion, cover, and cook until softened, about 5 minutes. Add the mushrooms and cook, uncovered, 5 minutes longer. Stir in the ginger and green onions. Add the tofu and soy sauce and cook until heated through, stirring to combine well, about 5 minutes. Stir in the cooked edamame and cook until heated through, about 5 minutes.

3. Divide the hot rice among 4 bowls, top each with the edamame and tofu mixture, and drizzle on the sesame oil. Sprinkle with sesame seeds and serve immediately.

Italian Wedding Soup

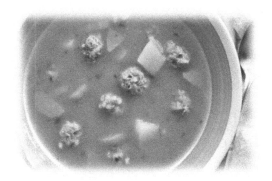

Preparation time: 10 minutes

Cooking time: 15 minutes

Servings: 4

Nutrition: (2 cups)

- Calories: 168
- Protein: 9g
- Total fat: 3g
- Saturated fat: 0g

- Carbohydrates: 30g
- Fiber: 6g

Ingredients:

- 1 teaspoon olive oil
- 2 carrots, peeled and chopped
- ½ onion, chopped
- 3 or 4 garlic cloves, minced, or ½ teaspoon garlic powder
- Salt
- 8 cups water or Economical Vegetable Broth
- 1 cup orzo or pearl couscous
- 1 tablespoon dried herbs
- Freshly ground black pepper
- 1 recipe quinoa meatballs
- 2 cups chopped greens, such as spinach, kale, or chard

Directions:

1. Heat the olive oil in a large soup pot over medium-high heat.
2. Add the carrots, onion, garlic (if using fresh), and a pinch of salt. Sauté for 3 to 4 minutes, until softened. Add the

water, orzo, and dried herbs (plus the garlic powder, if using). Season to taste with salt and pepper, and bring the soup to a boil. Turn the heat to low and simmer until the orzo is soft, about 10 minutes. Add the meatballs and greens, and stir until the greens are wilted. Taste and season with more salt and pepper as needed. Leftovers will keep in an airtight container for up to 1 week in the refrigerator or up to 1 month in the freezer.

Roasted Vegetable Bisque

Preparation time: 10 minutes

Cooking time: 15 minutes

Servings: 6

Ingredients:

- 1 large onion, coarsely chopped
- 2 medium carrots, coarsely chopped
- 1 large russet potato, peeled and cut into 1⁄2-inch dice
- 1 medium zucchini, thinly sliced
- 1 large ripe tomato, quartered
- 2 garlic cloves, crushed
- 2 tablespoons olive oil
- 1⁄2 teaspoon dried savory 1⁄2 teaspoon dried thyme
- Salt and freshly ground black pepper
- 4 cups vegetable broth (homemade, -bought, or water)
- 1 tablespoon minced fresh parsley, for garnish

Directions:

1. Preheat the oven to 400°F. In a lightly oiled 9 x 13-inch baking pan, place the onion, carrots, potato, zucchini, tomato, and garlic. Drizzle with the oil and season with savory, thyme, and salt and pepper to taste. Cover tightly with foil and bake until softened, about 30 minutes. Uncover and bake, stirring once, until vegetables are lightly browned, about 30 minutes more.

2. Transfer the roasted vegetables to a large soup pot, add the broth, and bring to a boil. Reduce the heat to low and simmer, uncovered, for 15 minutes.

3. Puree the soup in the pot with an immersion blender or in a blender or food processor, in batches if necessary, and return to the pot. Heat over medium heat until hot. Taste, adjusting seasonings if necessary.

4. Ladle into bowls, sprinkle with parsley, and serve.

Spicy Gazpacho

Preparation time: 15 minutes

Cooking time: 0 minutes

Servings: 4

Ingredients:

- 1 tablespoon olive oil
- 3 cups vegetable juice, such as v8
- 1 red onion, diced
- 3 tomatoes, chopped
- 1 red bell pepper, diced
- 2 garlic cloves, minced
- juice of 1 lemon
- 2 tablespoons chopped fresh basil
- ¼ to ½ teaspoon cayenne pepper sea salt
- freshly ground black pepper

Directions:

1. In a blender or a food processor, combine the olive oil, vegetable juice, all but ½ cup of the onion, all but ½ cup of the tomato, all but ½ cup of the bell pepper, the garlic, lemon juice, basil, and cayenne. Season with salt and pepper and process until smooth.
2. Stir the reserved ½ cup onion, ½ cup tomatoes, and ½ cup bell pepper into the processed ingredients and refrigerate for 1 hour. Serve chilled.

Parsley-Lime Pasta

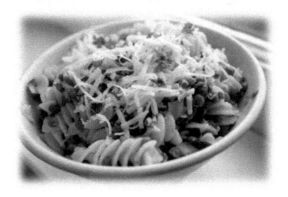

Preparation time: 20 minutes

Serving: 4

Nutritional Values (Per Serving):

- Calories: 326
- Total Fat: 24.9g
- Saturated Fat:12.9 g
- Total Carbs: 6 g
- Dietary Fiber:1g

- Sugar: 4g
- Protein: 20g
- Sodium: 568mg

Ingredients:

- 2 tbsp butter
- 1 lb tempeh, chopped
- 4 garlic cloves, minced
- 1 pinch red chili flakes
- ¼ cup white wine
- 1 lime, zested and juiced
- 3 medium zucchinis, spiralized
- Salt and black pepper to taste
- 2 tbsp chopped parsley
- 1 cup grated parmesan cheese for topping

Directions:

1. Melt the butter in a large skillet and cook in the tempeh until golden brown.
2. Flip and stir in the garlic and red chili flakes. Cook further for 1 minute; transfer to a plate and set aside.

3. Pour the wine and lime juice into the skillet, and cook until reduced by a quarter. Meanwhile, stir to deglaze the bottom of the pot.

4. Mix in the zucchinis, lime zest, tempeh and parsley. Season with salt and black pepper, and toss everything well. Cook until the zucchinis is slightly tender for 2 minutes.

5. Dish the food onto serving plates and top generously with the parmesan cheese.

Rice Salad with Cashews and Dried Papaya

Preparation time: 15 minutes

Cooking time: 0 minutes

Servings: 4

Ingredients:

- 3½ cups cooked brown rice
- ½ cup chopped roasted cashews
- ½ cup thinly sliced dried papaya
- 4 green onions, chopped
- 3 tablespoons fresh lime juice
- 2 teaspoons agave nectar
- 1 teaspoon grated fresh ginger
- ⅓ cup grapeseed oil
- Salt and freshly ground black pepper

Directions:

1. In a large bowl, combine the rice, cashews, papaya, and green onions. Set aside.

2. In a small bowl, combine the lime juice, agave nectar, and ginger. Whisk in the oil and season with the salt and pepper to taste. Pour the dressing over the rice mixture, mix well, and serve.

Spinach Salad with Orange-Dijon Dressing

Preparation time: 10 minutes

Cooking time: 0 minutes

Servings: 4

Ingredients:

- 2 tablespoons Dijon mustard
- 2 tablespoons olive oil
- 1⁄4 cup fresh orange juice
- 1 teaspoon agave nectar
- 1⁄2 teaspoon salt
- 1⁄4 teaspoon freshly ground black pepper
- 2 tablespoons minced fresh parsley
- 1 tablespoon minced green onions
- 5 cups fresh baby spinach, torn into bite-size pieces
- 1 navel orange, peeled and segmented
- 1⁄2 small red onion, sliced paper thin

Directions:

1. In a blender or food processor combine the mustard, oil, orange juice, agave nectar, salt, pepper, parsley, and green onions. Blend well and set aside.
2. In a large bowl, combine the spinach, orange, and onion. Add the dressing, toss gently to combine, and serve.

Caramelized Onion and Beet Salad

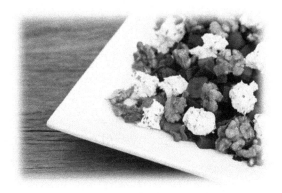

Preparation time: 10 minutes

Cooking time: 40 minutes

Servings: 4

Nutritional Values (Per Serving):

- Calories: 104
- Fat: 2g
- Protein: 3g
- Carbohydrates: 20g
- Fiber: 4g

- Sugar: 14g
- Sodium: 303mg

Ingredients:

- 3 medium golden beets
- 2 cups sliced sweet or Vidalia onions
- 1 teaspoon extra-virgin olive oil or no-beef broth
- Pinch baking soda
- ¼ to ½ teaspoon salt, to taste
- 2 tablespoons unseasoned rice vinegar, white wine vinegar, or balsamic vinegar

Directions:

1. Cut the greens off the beets, and scrub the beets.
2. In a large pot, place a steamer basket and fill the pot with 2 inches of water.
3. add the beets, bring to a boil, then reduce the heat to medium, cover, and steam for about 35 minutes, until you can easily pierce the middle of the beets with a knife.
4. Meanwhile, in a large, dry skillet over medium heat, sauté the onions for 5 minutes, stirring frequently.

5. Add the olive oil and baking soda, and continuing cooking for 5 more minutes, stirring frequently. Stir in the salt to taste before removing from the heat. Transfer to a large bowl and set aside.

6. When the beets have cooked through, drain and cool until easy to handle. Rub the beets in a paper towel to easily remove the skins. Cut into wedges, and transfer to the bowl with the onions. Drizzle the vinegar over everything and toss well.

7. Divide the beets evenly among 4 wide-mouth jars or storage containers. Let cool before sealing the lids.

Treasure Barley Salad

Preparation time: 10 minutes

Cooking time: 30 minutes

Servings: 4 to 6

Ingredients:

- 1 cup pearl barley
- 1½ cups cooked or 1 (15.5-ouncecan navy beans, drained and rinsed
- 1 celery rib, finely chopped
- 1 medium carrot, shredded
- 3 green onions, minced
- ½ cup chopped pitted kalamata olives
- ½ cup dried cherries or sweetened dried cranberries
- ½ cup toasted pecans pieces, coarsely chopped
- ½ cup minced fresh parsley
- 1 garlic clove, pressed
- 3 tablespoons sherry vinegar

- Salt and freshly ground black pepper
- 1⁄4 cup grapeseed oil

Directions:

1. In a large saucepan, bring 21⁄2 cups salted water to boil over high heat. Add the barley and return to a boil. Reduce heat to low, cover, and simmer until the barley is tender, about 30 minutes. Transfer to a serving bowl.
2. Add the beans, celery, carrot, green onions, olives, cherries, pecans, and parsley. Set aside.
3. In a small bowl, combine the garlic, vinegar, and salt and pepper to taste. Whisk in the oil until well blended. Pour the dressing over the salad, toss to combine, and serve.

Garden Salad Wraps

Preparation time: 15 minutes

Cooking time: 10 minutes

Servings: 4 wraps

Ingredients:

- 6 tablespoons olive oil
- 1 pound extra-firm tofu, drained, patted dry, and cut into 1⁄2-inch strips
- 1 tablespoon soy sauce
- 1⁄4 cup apple cider vinegar
- 1 teaspoon yellow or spicy brown mustard
- 1⁄2 teaspoon salt
- 1⁄4 teaspoon freshly ground black pepper
- 3 cups shredded romaine lettuce
- 3 ripe Roma tomatoes, finely chopped
- 1 large carrot, shredded

- 1 medium English cucumber, peeled and chopped
- 1⁄3 cup minced red onion
- 1⁄4 cup sliced pitted green olives
- 4 (10-inchwhole-grain flour tortillas or lavash flatbread

Directions:

1. In a large skillet, heat 2 tablespoons of the oil over medium heat. Add the tofu and cook until golden brown, about 10 minutes. Sprinkle with soy sauce and set aside to cool.
2. In a small bowl, combine the vinegar, mustard, salt, and pepper with the remaining 4 tablespoons oil, stirring to blend well. Set aside.
3. In a large bowl, combine the lettuce, tomatoes, carrot, cucumber, onion, and olives. Pour on the dressing and toss to coat.
4. To assemble wraps, place 1 tortilla on a work surface and spread with about one-quarter of the salad. Place a few strips of tofu on the tortilla and roll up tightly. Slice in half

Black Sesame Wonton Chips

Preparation time: 5 minutes

Cooking time: 5 minutes

Servings: 24 chips

Ingredients:

- 12 Vegan Wonton Wrappers
- Toasted sesame oil
- 1/3 cup black sesame seeds
- Salt

Directions:

1. Preheat the oven to 450°F. Lightly oil a baking sheet and set aside. Cut the wonton wrappers in half crosswise, brush them with sesame oil, and arrange them in a single layer on the prepared baking sheet.
2. Sprinkle wonton wrappers with the sesame seeds and salt to taste, and bake until crisp and golden brown, 5 to 7

minutes. Cool completely before serving. These are best eaten on the day they are made but, once cooled, they can be covered and stored at room temperature for 1 to 2 days.

Marinated Mushroom Wraps

Preparation time: 15 minutes

Cooking time: 0 minutes

Servings: 2 wraps

Ingredients:

- 3 tablespoons soy sauce
- 3 tablespoons fresh lemon juice
- 1½ tablespoons toasted sesame oil
- 2 portobello mushroom caps, cut into ¼-inch strips
- 1 ripe Hass avocado, pitted and peeled
- 2 (10-inchwhole-grain flour tortillas
- 2 cups fresh baby spinach leaves
- 1 medium red bell pepper, cut into ¼-inch strips
- 1 ripe tomato, chopped
- Salt and freshly ground black pepper

Directions:

In a medium bowl, combine the soy sauce, 2 tablespoons of the lemon juice, and the oil. Add the portobello strips, toss to combine, and marinate for 1 hour or overnight. Drain the mushrooms and set aside.

Mash the avocado with the remaining 1 tablespoon of lemon juice.

To assemble wraps, place 1 tortilla on a work surface and spread with some of the mashed avocado. Top with a layer of baby spinach leaves. In the lower third of each tortilla, arrange strips of the soaked mushrooms and some of the bell pepper strips. Sprinkle with the tomato and salt and black pepper to taste. Roll up tightly and cut in half diagonally. Repeat with the remaining ingredients and serve.

Tamari Toasted Almonds

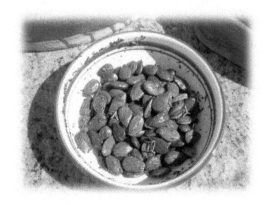

Preparation time: 2 minutes

Cooking time: 8 minutes

Servings: ½ cup

Nutrition (1 tablespoon)

- Calories: 89
- Total fat: 8g
- Carbs: 3g
- Fiber: 2g
- Protein: 4g

Ingredients:

- ½ cup raw almonds, or sunflower seeds
- 2 tablespoons tamari, or soy sauce
- 1 teaspoon toasted sesame oil

Directions:

1. Heat a dry skillet to medium-high heat, then add the almonds, stirring very frequently to keep them from burning. Once the almonds are toasted, 7 to 8 minutes for almonds, or 3 to 4 minutes for sunflower seeds, pour the tamari and sesame oil into the hot skillet and stir to coat.
2. You can turn off the heat, and as the almonds cool the tamari mixture will stick to and dry on the nuts.

Avocado and Tempeh Bacon Wraps

Preparation time: 10 minutes

Cooking time: 8 minutes

Servings: 4 wraps

Ingredients:

- 2 tablespoons olive oil
- 8 ounces tempeh bacon, homemade or store-bought
- 4 (10-inchsoft flour tortillas or lavash flat bread
- 1/4 cup vegan mayonnaise, homemade or store-bought
- 4 large lettuce leaves
- 2 ripe Hass avocados, pitted, peeled, and cut into 1/4-inch slices
- 1 large ripe tomato, cut into 1/4-inch slices

Directions:

In a large skillet, heat the oil over medium heat. Add the tempeh bacon and cook until browned on both sides, about 8 minutes. Remove from the heat and set aside.

Place 1 tortilla on a work surface. Spread with some of the mayonnaise and one-fourth of the lettuce and tomatoes.

Pit, peel, and thinly slice the avocado and place the slices on top of the tomato. Add the reserved tempeh bacon and roll up tightly. Repeat with remaining ingredients and serve.

Cherry-Vanilla Rice Pudding (Pressure cooker)

Preparation time: 5 minutes

Servings: 4-6

Nutrition:

- Calories: 177
- Total fat: 1g
- Protein: 3g
- Sodium: 27mg
- Fiber: 2g

Ingredients:

- 1 cup short-grain brown rice
- 1¾ cups nondairy milk, plus more as needed

- 1½ cups water
- 4 tablespoons unrefined sugar or pure maple syrup (use 2 tablespoons if you use a sweetened milk), plus more as needed
- 1 teaspoon vanilla extract (use ½ teaspoon if you use vanilla milk
- Pinch salt
- ¼ cup dried cherries or ½ cup fresh or frozen pitted cherries

Directions:

1. In your electric pressure cooker's cooking pot, combine the rice, milk, water, sugar, vanilla, and salt.
2. High pressure for 30 minutes. Close and lock the lid and ensure the pressure valve is sealed, then select High Pressure and set the time for 30 minutes.
3. Pressure Release. Once the cook time is complete, let the pressure release naturally, about 20 minutes. Once all the pressure has released, carefully unlock and remove the lid. Stir in the cherries and put the lid back on loosely for about 10 minutes. Serve, adding more milk or sugar, as desired.

Chocolate Coconut Brownies

Preparation time: 5 minutes

Cooking time: 35 minutes

Servings: 12 brownies

Ingredients:

- 1 cup whole-grain flour
- 1/2 cup unsweetened cocoa powder
- 1 teaspoon baking powder
- 1/2 teaspoon salt
- 1 cup light brown sugar
- 1/2 cup canola oil
- 3/4 cup unsweetened coconut milk
- 1 teaspoon pure vanilla extract
- 1 teaspoon coconut extract
- 1/2 cup vegan semisweet chocolate chips
- 1/2 cup sweetened shredded coconut

Directions:

1. Preheat the oven to 350°F. Grease an 8-inch square baking pan and set aside. In a large bowl, combine the flour, cocoa, baking powder, and salt. Set aside.
2. In a medium bowl, mix together the sugar and oil until blended. Stir in the coconut milk
3. and the extracts and blend until smooth. Add the wet ingredients to the dry ingredients: stirring to blend. Fold in the chocolate chips and coconut.
4. Scrape the batter into the prepared baking pan and bake until the center is set and a toothpick inserted in the center comes out clean, 35 to 40 minutes. Let the brownies cool 30 minutes before serving. Store in an airtight container.

Lime in the Coconut Chia Pudding

Preparation time: 10 minutes • chill time: 20 minutes

Servings: 4

Nutrition:

- Calories: 226
- Total fat: 20g
- Carbs: 13g
- Fiber: 5g
- Protein: 3g

Ingredients:

- Zest and juice of 1 lime
- 1 (14-ouncecan coconut milk
- 1 to 2 dates, or 1 tablespoon coconut or other unrefined
  sugar, or 1 tablespoon maple syrup, or 10 to 15 drops pure
  liquid stevia

- 2 tablespoons chia seeds, whole or ground
- 2 teaspoons matcha green tea powder (optional

Directions:

1. Blend all the ingredients in a blender until smooth. Chill in the fridge for about 20 minutes, then serve topped with one or more of the topping ideas.
2. Try blueberries, blackberries, sliced strawberries, Coconut Whipped Cream, or toasted unsweetened coconut.

Strawberry Parfaits with Cashew Crème

Preparation time: 10 minutes • chill time: 50 minutes •

Servings: 4

Ingredients:

- ½ cup unsalted raw cashews
- 4 tablespoons light brown sugar
- ½ cup plain or vanilla soy milk
- ¾ cup firm silken tofu, drained
- 1 teaspoon pure vanilla extract
- 2 cups sliced strawberries
- 1 teaspoon fresh lemon juice
- Fresh mint leaves, for garnish

Directions:

1. In a blender, grind the cashews and 3 tablespoons of the sugar to a fine powder. Add the soy milk and blend until

smooth. Add the tofu and vanilla and continue to blend until smooth and creamy. Scrape the cashew mixture into a medium bowl, cover, and refrigerate for 30 minutes.

2. In a large bowl, combine the strawberries, lemon juice, and remaining 1 tablespoon sugar. Stir gently to combine and set aside at room temperature for 20 minutes.

3. Spoon alternating layers of the strawberries and cashew crème into parfait glasses or wineglasses, ending with a dollop of the cashew crème. Garnish with mint leaves and serve.

Mint Chocolate Chip Sorbet

Preparation time: 5 minutes

Cooking time: 0 minutes

Servings: 1

Nutrition:

- Calories: 212
- Total fat: 10g
- Carbs: 31g
- Fiber: 4g
- Protein: 3g

Ingredients:

- 1 frozen banana
- 1 tablespoon almond butter, or peanut butter, or other nut or seed butter
- 2 tablespoons fresh mint, minced
- ¼ cup or less non-dairy milk (only if needed)

- 2 to 3 tablespoons non-dairy chocolate chips, or cocoa nibs
- 2 to 3 tablespoons goji berries (optional)

Directions:

1. Put the banana, almond butter, and mint in a food processor or blender and purée until smooth.
2. Add the non-dairy milk if needed to keep blending (but only if needed, as this will make the texture less solid). Pulse the chocolate chips and goji berries (if usinginto the mix so they're roughly chopped up.

Peach-Mango Crumble (Pressure cooker)

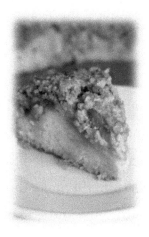

Preparation time: 10 minutes

Servings: 4-6

Nutrition:

- Calories: 321
- Total fat: 18g
- Protein: 4g
- Sodium: 2mg
- Fiber: 7g

Ingredients:

- 3 cups chopped fresh or frozen peaches
- 3 cups chopped fresh or frozen mangos
- 4 tablespoons unrefined sugar or pure maple syrup, divided
- 1 cup gluten-free rolled oats
- ½ cup shredded coconut, sweetened or unsweetened
- 2 tablespoons coconut oil or vegan margarine

Directions:

1. In a 6- to 7-inch round baking dish, toss together the peaches, mangos, and 2 tablespoons of sugar. In a food processor, combine the oats, coconut, coconut oil, and remaining 2 tablespoons of sugar. Pulse until combined. (If you use maple syrup, you'll need less coconut oil. Start with just the syrup and add oil if the mixture isn't sticking together. Sprinkle the oat mixture over the fruit mixture.

2. Cover the dish with aluminum foil. Put a trivet in the bottom of your electric pressure cooker's cooking pot and pour in a cup or two of water. Using a foil sling or silicone helper handles, lower the pan onto the trivet.

3. High pressure for 6 minutes. Close and lock the lid and ensure the pressure valve is sealed, then select High Pressure and set the time for 6 minutes.

4. Pressure Release. Once the cook time is complete, quick release the pressure, being careful not to get your fingers or face near the steam release. Once all the pressure has released, carefully unlock and remove the lid.

5. Let cool for a few minutes before carefully lifting out the dish with oven mitts or tongs. Scoop out portions to serve.

Ginger-Spice Brownies

Preparation time: 5 minutes

Cooking time: 35 minutes

Servings: 12 brownies

Ingredients:

- 1¾ cups whole-grain flour
- 1 teaspoon baking powder
- 1 teaspoon baking soda
- ½ teaspoon salt
- 1 tablespoon ground ginger
- ½ teaspoon ground cinnamon
- ½ teaspoon ground allspice
- 3 tablespoons unsweetened cocoa powder
- ½ cup vegan semisweet chocolate chips
- ½ cup chopped walnuts
- ¼ cup canola oil
- ½ cup dark molasses
- ½ cup water

- 1/3 cup light brown sugar
- 2 teaspoons grated fresh ginger

Directions:

1. Preheat the oven to 350°F. Grease an 8-inch square baking pan and set aside. In a large bowl, combine the flour, baking powder, baking soda, salt, ground ginger, cinnamon, allspice, and cocoa. Stir in the chocolate chips and walnuts and set aside.

2. In medium bowl, combine the oil, molasses, water, sugar, and fresh ginger and mix well.

3. Pour the wet ingredients into the dry ingredients and mix well.

4. Scrape the dough into the prepared baking pan. The dough will be sticky, so wet your hands to press it evenly into the pan. Bake until a toothpick inserted in the center comes out clean, 30 to 35 minutes. Cool on a wire rack 30 minutes before cutting. Store in an airtight container.

Chocolate and Walnut Farfalle

Preparation time: 10 minutes

Cooking time: 0 minutes

Servings: 4

Ingredients:

- ½ cup chopped toasted walnuts
- ¼ cup vegan semisweet chocolate pieces
- 8 ounces farfalle
- 3 tablespoons vegan margarine
- ¼ cup ight brown sugar

Directions:

1. In a food processor or blender, grind the walnuts and chocolate pieces until crumbly. Do not overprocess. Set aside.

2. In a pot of boiling salted water, cook the farfalle, stirring occasionally, until al dente, about 8 minutes. Drain well and return to the pot.

3. Add the margarine and sugar and toss to combine and melt the margarine.

4. Transfer the noodle mixture to a serving.

Almond-Date Energy Bites

Preparation time: 5 minutes • chill time: 15 minutes

Servings: 24 bites

Nutrition (1 bite):

- Calories: 152
- Total fat: 11g
- Carbs: 13g
- Fiber: 5g
- Protein: 3g

Ingredients:

- 1 cup dates, pitted
- 1 cup unsweetened shredded coconut
- ¼ cup chia seeds
- ¾ cup ground almonds
- ¼ cup cocoa nibs, or non-dairy chocolate chips

Directions:

1. Purée everything in a food processor until crumbly and sticking together, pushing down the sides whenever necessary to keep it blending. If you don't have a food processor, you can mash soft Medjool dates. But if you're using harder baking dates, you'll have to soak them and then try to purée them in a blender.

2. Form the mix into 24 balls and place them on a baking sheet lined with parchment or waxed paper. Put in the fridge to set for about 15 minutes. Use the softest dates you can find. Medjool dates are the best for this purpose. The hard dates you see in the baking aisle of your supermarket are going to take a long time to blend up. If you use those, try soaking them in water for at least an hour before you start, and then draining.

Cloud Bread

Preparation time: 15 minutes

Cooking time: 35 minutes

Servings: 6

Nutritions:

- Calories 82
- Fat 7g
- Protein 4g
- Carbs 1g
- Fiber 0g
- Sugar 0g
- Sodium 123mg

Ingredients:

- Nonstick cooking spray
- 3 eggs, separated, at room temperature
- 3 ounces cream cheese, at room temperature
- ⅛ teaspoon salt

Directions:

1. Preheat the oven to 300°F. Spray a baking sheet with cooking spray.
2. In a large mixing bowl, use a handheld electric mixer to beat the egg whites into stiff peaks. Set aside.
3. In a separate large bowl, combine the egg yolks, cream cheese, and salt, and mix until creamy.
4. Slowly pour the egg white mixture into the egg yolk mixture, and use a spatula to carefully fold it in. Be careful not to overmix.
5. Use the batter to make 6 separate circles on the prepared baking sheet. These will be your clouds.
6. Bake for 30 to 35 minutes or until golden brown.
7. Remove from the oven and allow to cool for 10 minutes before serving.

Fathead Crackers

Preparation time: 15 minutes

Cooking time: 10 minutes

Servings: 4

Nutritions:

- Calories 225
- Fat 18g
- Protein 13g
- Carbs 3g
- Fiber 1g
- Sugar 1g
- Sodium 591mg

Ingredients:

- Nonstick cooking spray
- 1½ cups grated mozzarella cheese
- ⅔ cup almond flour

- 2 tablespoons cream cheese
- 1 egg
- ½ teaspoon salt

Directions:

1. Preheat the oven to 425°F. Spray a baking sheet with cooking spray.
2. In a microwave-safe bowl, combine the mozzarella, almond flour, and cream cheese.
3. Microwave on high for 1 minute. Remove carefully and stir, then cook for an additional 30 seconds.
4. Remove the bowl and add the egg and salt. Stir quickly until a ball of dough forms.
5. Roll out the dough to ¼-inch thick. Olive oil can be used to avoid sticking.
6. Cut the dough into 1-inch squares. Use a spatula to carefully transfer the crackers to the prepared baking sheet.
7. Cook for 5 minutes. Flip and cook for another 5 minutes.
8. Transfer the crackers to a wire rack to cool.

Queso Blanco Dip

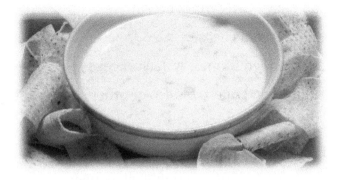

Preparation time: 5 minutes

Cooking time: 10 minutes

Servings: 8

Nutritions:

- Calories 202
- Fat 18g
- Protein 8g
- Carbs 2g
- Fiber 0g
- Sugar 1g
- Sodium 265mg

Ingredients:

- ½ cup heavy (whipping) cream
- 3 ounces cream cheese
- 1 cup shredded Monterey Jack cheese
- 1 cup shredded queso blanco or other sharp white cheddar cheese
- 1 (4.5-ounce) can diced green chiles, drained
- ½ teaspoon freshly ground black pepper
- ½ teaspoon ground cumin

Directions:

1. In a small saucepan over medium heat, melt together the heavy cream and cream cheese, whisking until totally melted.
2. Stir in the Monterey Jack cheese and queso blanco and the green chiles.
3. Remove from the heat and add the pepper and cumin.
4. Stir well and serve.

Classic Buttermilk Syrup

Preparation time: 5 minutes

Cooking time: 10 minutes

Servings: 12

Nutritions:

- Calories 137
- Fat 15g
- Protein 0g
- Carbs 0g
- Fiber 0g
- Sugar 0g
- Sodium 133mg
- Erythritol Carbs 16g

Ingredients:

- ¾ cup grass-fed butter
- ½ cup heavy (whipping) cream

- ¾ teaspoon white distilled vinegar
- ¼ cup water
- 1 cup powdered monk fruit
- ⅛ teaspoon salt
- 1 teaspoon baking soda
- 1 teaspoon vanilla extract

Directions:

1. In a large saucepan over medium heat, melt the butter.
2. In a small bowl, mix together the heavy cream and vinegar. Allow to sit for 5 minutes.
3. Add the water and monk fruit to the butter, whisking until all the sweetener has dissolved.
4. Add the cream mixture and salt to the pan, continuing to whisk while bringing the mixture to a gentle boil.
5. Remove the pan from the heat and stir in the baking soda and vanilla. Keep an eye on it because it will foam up. Whisk until all the foam is gone.
6. Serve warm.

Baked Onion Rings

Preparation time: 5 minutes

Cooking time: 25 minutes

Servings: 4

Nutritions:

- Calories: 130
- Carbohydrates: 10.7 G
- Fat: 7.4 G
- Sugar: 3.5 G
- Cholesterol: 82 Mg
- Protein: 6.1 G

Ingredients:

- 2 eggs, organic
- ½ teaspoon pepper
- ½ teaspoon salt
- ½ teaspoon garlic powder

- 2 tablespoons thyme, sliced
- 1 ½ cups almond flour
- 2 large sweet onions, cut into rings

Directions:

1. Preheat your oven to 400° fahrenheit. In a mixing bowl, combine garlic powder, almond flour, thyme, garlic powder, and salt. Take another bowl, add eggs and whisk. Dip the onion ring in egg mixture then coat with flour mixture. Place the coated onion rings in a baking dish. Bake in preheated oven for 25 minutes. Serve immediately and enjoy!

Lightning Source UK Ltd.
Milton Keynes UK
UKHW020628060521
383207UK00003B/283